"*The husband and wife co-authors offer a u[nique?]* [...] *disorder that is both interesting and inspiring. L[...] practical information and motivate them to take control of their health.*

> ~ Peggy McColl
> *New York Times* Bestselling Author

"*Jenna Michaud-Bonyadi has written a masterpiece... Incredibly comprehensive, insightful, and progressive; this is an invaluable tool for navigating the complexities of TMJ dysfunction, and finding your way back to pain-free living.*"

> ~ Joy Walraven, R. Ac., R. TCMP, CST
> Acupuncture, Traditional Chinese Medicine, Craniosacral Therapy

"*Suffering from TMJ disorder can have debilitating effects on people's lives. This book truly is a roadmap to helping anyone suffering with this type of pain. Dr. and Mrs Bonyadi have used scientific as well as real-life methods for relieving this disorder. I plan on using these methods for my own patients!*"

> ~ Stephanie Aldrich DDS FAGD FICOI, author of "Nothing But the Tooth – 11 Questions You Should Ask Your Dentist"

"*From my own experiences as a patient, I can so relate to natural approaches to resolving TMJ disorder. I was so taken by surprise someone would have the guts to write such a book as this alternative roadmap. It is very commendable... as well as inspiring!*

> ~ Callie K LeVina

"*Jenna and Dino have made the confusing causes and treatment options of TMJ, simple and practical to navigate through. Great job!!!*"

> ~ Anthony B. Morovati, DC
> Diplomate, American Academy of Pain Management

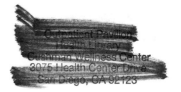

Published by
Hasmark Publishing
www.hasmarkpublishing.com

Disclaimer

This book is designed to provide information and motivation to our readers. It is sold with the understanding that the publisher is not engaged to render any type of psychological, legal, or any other kind of professional advice. The content of each article is the sole expression and opinion of its author, and not necessarily that of the publisher. No warranties or guarantees are expressed or implied by the publisher's choice to include any of the content in this volume. Neither the publisher nor the individual author(s) shall be liable for any physical, psychological, emotional, financial, or commercial damages, including, but not limited to, special, incidental, consequential or other damages. Our views and rights are the same: You are responsible for your own choices, actions, and results.

Permission should be addressed in writing to Jenna Michaud-Bonyadi and Dino Bonyadi, DDS at jenna@tmjroadmap.com or by mail to 1315 S. Miller St., #201, Santa Maria California 93454

Editor: Sigrid Macdonald
Book Magic
http://bookmagic.biz

Cover Designer & Layout Artist: Anne Karklins
annekarklins@gmail.com

ISBN 13: 978-1-989161-35-7
ISBN 10: 1989161359

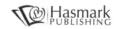

Your R⊕admap to TMJ Health

How to Navigate Your Way Through TMJ Disorder
with a Comprehensive Approach to Healing

JENNA MICHAUD-BONYADI
and **DINO BONYADI** DDS

*This book is dedicated to everyone searching for a
path to wellness, especially those with chronic pain conditions.
To anyone with TMJD, this book is for you.*

Acknowledgements

The authors would like to thank all those who supported and participated in the creation of this book. First, all of the people living with TMJD who opened their hearts and shared their stories in an effort to help others. Your individual perspectives helped to shed light on both the similarities and differences that exist in everyone's unique experience of TMJD. Thank you to the healthcare providers who, by giving their time and sharing their expertise, confirmed the core purpose of this book. With special thanks to the caring hearts of Dr. Anthony B. Morovati, DC, Dr. Anthony Pitrowski, DMD, MD, OMFS, and Dr. Eric Minassian, DC. Our eternal gratitude must go to Peggy McColl. Without her expert guidance, this book would still be locked up inside the hearts and minds of the authors.

I would like to thank Stanford University School of Medicine for their study on love and pain. I would also like to thank The National Institute of Dental and Craniofacial Research for their information regarding the study of direct neurological connections between pain above the neck and the fear/anxiety center of the brain.

Table of Contents

Section 1: Introduction   9

My Story   11

Why you need a roadmap   13

How to use this book   17

Section 2: Understanding TMJ Disorder   21

Basic Anatomy of the Human Jaw   23

What is TMJ Disorder – Definitions, Symptoms, & Causes   24

**Section 3: Assemble Your Dream Team! A team approach to   35
TMJ health and putting together your team of healers.**

Why You Need a Team of Healers.   37

Where to Begin. Your first step on the road to TMJ health.   41

What role each team member plays on the road to TMJ health.   46

MD/Family Physician   47

Dentist   48

Chiropractor   50

Physical Therapy   51

Acupuncture, Massage & Bodywork   51

Non-Physical Approaches   53

Self-Care   54

Section 4: Destination – TMJ Health!   57

What To Do Next   59

Self Assessment "You Are Here" (Worksheet 1)   61

Keep Going (Worksheet 2)   67

"Quality of Life Goals" (Worksheet 2)   69

Roadmap Builder   75

Circle of Wellness   76

Interview Questions   77

Wellness Pledge   79

Wellness Journal   80

SECTION 1

Introduction

My Story

I have been living with TMJ disorder for most of my life. In fact, I was probably born with it. That's close to 45 years as of the writing of this book. One of the first signs was that as a child, I would eat very slowly, likely due to the fact that my jaw was not functioning properly. Later as a teenager I began experiencing "clicking" sounds in my jaw. At the time, I thought it was just one of the idiosyncrasies that made me "me". Like being so-called "double jointed" in my arms and hands, I thought my jaw joint was a little different than most, but that it was nothing to be concerned about. I had no idea this was a sign of a problem that would lead to pain and discomfort later in life. Fast forward to my college years when the jaw pain really began. I remember sitting in lectures and using a highlighter pen to try to rub away the soreness in my jaw joint. Surely, this was distracting me and I wasn't even aware at the time. Like many who suffer from TMJ related pain and discomfort, the symptoms had come on slowly over a long period of time , so it was not as noticeable as experiencing that level of pain right from the get go. The joint on the right side of my jaw was degrading and would soon cause me terrible headaches, muscle fatigue when speaking and eating, difficulty chewing, as well as neck and shoulder pain. I remember times when my jaw would suddenly lock up and really scare me because I couldn't open or close it at all. The muscle fatigue would cause me to slur my words or speak in a strange manner because of the need to almost force my jaw into positions it didn't want to go into but that are needed for speech. There was a time I felt hopeless and that I would just have to live with the pain and dysfunction that would continue to worsen over time.

The frightening advice I received from some doctors a few years later did not give me hope for healing or recovery of any sort. In effect they basically told me my pain and suffering would worsen and I would probably need surgery and/or extreme dental procedures later in life. At my lowest point, I felt like I was truly disabled. I remember sitting at the kitchen table as tears fell into my bowl of soup, feeling like a freak that would ONLY be able to eat soup for the rest of her life. And my case was not even very severe in relation to how bad it can be for many people living with TMJ disorder. Along my journey to a healthy TMJ and during my research for writing this book, I became aware of the fact that there are many people with far worse cases than mine. I can tell you that today I am pain free and my TMJ does not impact my quality of life in a negative way. Also, I eat more than just soup.

The second part of my story is that I met and married a dentist. My husband and co-author of this book is Dino Bonyadi, DDS and he is a general dentist. We did not meet because of my TMJ problem; actually, it's the other way around. He was in dental school when we met, so he was not treating me or seeing me as a patient. I was in my 20s and, in fact, up to this point, I had sought no treatment for it at all. However, due to my suffering from the worsening symptoms of TMJ disorder, my husband began to study extensively on the subject in order to help me. As a new graduate from the University of Southern California School of Dentistry in 1992, he was passionate about wanting to help me. It is this journey as husband and wife as well as doctor and patient that we share with you here in this book. We are still married today (26 years later) and as I said before, I am TMJ pain free. Along the way, we learned and tried many different approaches to help me be more comfortable. We tried pretty much everything except surgery. Some things helped and others did not. The specialists who scared me with their opinions about needing surgery were some of the other doctors we consulted along the way. Fortunately, we followed our instincts to try everything non-invasive first in the hopes of avoiding surgery and other extreme and/or invasive measures. Additionally, my husband employed what he learned about TMJ disorder in his private practice to help his other patients. Over time we began to see how many other people were suffering like I was or even more so. Also, we saw how misunderstood the problem was and that a comprehensive approach was needed. Dino felt that it was difficult to communicate everything he wanted to his patients about TMJ disorder in just a short exam time. TMJ disorder patients needed more knowledge and education than is possible during a typical single exam with any doctor. We realized that we could help so many people by sharing the information we had learned. We decided to write this book in order to provide the information and guidance we felt TMJ disorder patients really needed.

I decided to share not only my story, but the stories of other people living with TMJ disorder since every case is different and there are various levels of dysfunction. My desire is that everyone who reads this book will benefit from it in some way. That is also why we have included the perspectives of several other health professionals and not just Dino's perspective as a general dentist. This includes several types of doctors and other healers. Please refer to Section 3 for a list of all the doctor and healer types. In order to present a comprehensive approach to treating TMJ disorder, all potential treatment options are considered here. Every treatment option is not right for every person who suffers from TMJ disorder. That is where you come in. As you navigate this road, you will plot your course with the help of the information provided in this book. It's up to you to discover what resources are readily available to you in your part of the world. By that I mean, to seek out and find your TMJ health "dream team" members. They are out there; you just have to know what to look for . This is great news because it means you are in control! It is also up to you to get to know yourself, so you can be an advocate for your own health. Armed with this information, you may put together a dream team of healers that also includes you! In fact, you will be the leader of this dream team.

My desire is for you to feel empowered to take control of your TMJ health. Actually, much of what is presented in this book can be applied to any health problem and I hope what you learn here will overflow into other areas of your life to the benefit of your overall health.

Why you need a roadmap

Pain of the face and head is especially debilitating. This is not just my opinion or the opinion of people suffering from TMJD. It is a scientific fact that we have twice the neural pathways from pain sensors in the head to the brain and spinal cord than from the rest of the body. Not only that but recent studies have shown one of the pathways is directly wired to a part of the brain responsible for a strong emotional fear response. If you have ever felt like you were crazy for the way your TMJD made you feel emotionally, this could be why. This is also why it can be hard for people close to a TMJD patient to understand their situation. Many people with orofacial pain like TMJD, migraines, cluster headaches, and so on are misunderstood and judged regarding how debilitating their pain is. If you have ever been perceived to be "overreacting" to your TMJD related pain, it is because the same level of pain in your hand or leg, for example, does not induce the same emotional fear response. That fear response, especially if not understood, can lead to anxiety and depression. Living in a heightened state of fear and anxiety, that "fight or flight" response is not healthy and can lead to a whole host of systemic illnesses. The National Institute of Health reports that "Studies have found that people rate head and facial pain as more severe, emotionally draining, and scary than pain elsewhere in the body." This, of course, applies to those suffering from migraines, cluster headaches, and any other pain of the head and face. TMJD patients often have a collection of more than one type of orofacial pain such as headaches along with jaw pain. When you are in a desperate state of pain- based fear and anxiety, it is very difficult to make good decisions. The goal of this book is to help ground you, so you can make decisions from a place of thoughtfulness. To help you go from just reacting to thinking and responding.

If you suffer from TMJ disorder and you are reading this book, most likely you have experienced sitting in your dentist's chair with a blank stare while he or she attempted to explain to you the causes and effects of your malady. Not all doctors are blessed with excellent communication skills and even if they are, they were trained to understand and communicate their knowledge with technical terms which often are not understood by their patients. Some doctors are skilled at being able to translate their technical knowledge into layman's terms. Others are not. This can leave you feeling lost and confused despite your doctor's best efforts to explain things to you.

There are plenty of scientific articles and journals on the subject of TMJ disorder and related jaw pain as well as treatment. However, they are usually written by doctors for other doctors. Such information is often focused on one specific type of treatment or another as in the results of a scientific study or research. So while the information is out there, it is not easily accessible to the layperson who has little to no knowledge of scientific or medical terminology. And even if you could extract some useful information out of technical resources, you would not have any idea how to put it to use for yourself.

We set out to write this book in order to present this information on navigating through TMJ disorder in an understandable and practical way, so that you may improve your quality of life as quickly as possible. Basic anatomy diagrams are included and structures defined to help you understand your body, more specifically your jaw joint, its function and related areas of concern. However, I will break everything down, so that it is understandable to practically anyone who can read.

Another reason that having a roadmap will help you to get positive results is this: The information needed to improve your situation can be overwhelming if presented in a way where everything is thrown at you all at once. It's almost impossible for anyone to fully hear, understand, and absorb all the necessary information in one or even a few sittings as is usually the case during typical doctor visits. Some people may feel intimidated by their doctor's education, but that's not the reason why you may have a hard time remembering and understanding things. It's not because you are not intelligent or "not as smart as the doctor". No, it is a fact of human learning. Neuroscientists estimate that within one hour, you will forget 50% of what you heard. Within 24 hours, you will forget 70% of the information and, within a week, 90% of the new information will be forgotten. It is incredibly helpful to have the information available in an organized way, so you can digest it little by little at your own pace. This way you can make a plan, step by step, and refer back to it when needed.

Moreover, each healthcare practitioner naturally approaches treatment of a medical problem from the perspective of his or her specialty. If you arbitrarily seek help from one type of doctor or healer over another, you are likely to get an opinion skewed in favor of the type of medicine he or she practices. The type of medicine they practice is the way they know how to help you. Those are the tools in their toolbox. For example, a dentist will likely suggest dental treatment options and a chiropractor will suggest chiropractic treatment options as a solution to your TMJ problem. It's not always intentional that most doctors don't embrace a multidisciplinary approach. It could be lack of interest in or knowledge on the subject of TMJ disorder, or it could be simply lack of experience and or exposure to TMJ disorders. The bottom line is this – if you only seek treatment from one type of doctor or healer, and do nothing else, you will not maximize your healing potential. In fact, the symptoms of your TMJ disorder could even increase. This is why so many people go around in circles in an attempt to alleviate their TMJ pain and may come to the conclusion that nothing works. You may have even tried more than one of the treatment options presented in this book. If you feel they failed you in the past or only helped temporarily, reconsider them in conjunction with other additional options this time. Also, reconsider having the same treatment provided by some-one else. The practitioner who performs the treatment is just as important as the treatment itself. Remember, there is no silver bullet or one magic device that will "cure" your TMJ disorder.

This leads me to another important point and motivation for writing this book. There is blatant misinformation out there, some of which can cost people to waste thousands of dollars. Some misinformation may not cost you much money, but could cost you time or cause you confusion. Worst of all, in my opinion, is the misinformation that causes someone additional pain and/or trauma either physical or mental/emotional. The core purpose of this book is to be a legitimate source of help for you to improve your quality of life by reducing TMJ associated pain. Truly, to help you create your roadmap to TMJ health.

Another maze to navigate through is that there is no approved standard of care for treating TMJ disorder and there is no medical specialty approved to treat TMJD specifically. Currently, there is no "TMJ doctor", so to speak. Clinics or doctors claiming to specialize in TMJ disorder have simply chosen to focus their area of practice on that subject and may have studied a certain technique or developed their own techniques regarding TMJD treatment. However, there is no "Board Certified" specialty like there is for ear/nose/throat doctors or an oral surgeon or endodontist, for example. Much of what is presented by such practices is experimental in nature. Could you get good results from treatment there? Sure, possibly. This book does not promote or oppose any specific treatment or product. The point is for you to be educated, aware, and know what you are choosing and why when you make a decision.

Finally, if you have found a doctor who embraces a multidisciplinary approach to treating your TMJ disorder, you are on the right track and should consider yourself very fortunate! If not, then don't worry as we will help you take the steps to put together your healing team.

One thing I have heard again and again when conducting interviews was how important it is for people living with TMJ disorder to know they are not alone. So, as mentioned before, I have included other people's stories and perspectives throughout the book. They are people who have "been down this road". Rest assured you are not alone, both from the healer/doctor viewpoint and from the patient viewpoint. This book is both evidence that you are not alone and a tool to help you surround yourself with a support network. I conducted interviews with patients and health-care providers because I truly believe we can always learn from looking at a situation from a different perspective. I felt that gathering together the experiences and knowledge of others would allow for a more well-rounded understanding of your own situation. Finally, using the experiences of myself and others will hopefully help you relate to the information on a personal level.

This roadmap is not only a practical tool to guide you toward TMJ health and the specific goals you have for that, but a source to provide you hope. For without hope, the power of your mind and emotions cannot be harnessed to set your intentions. Please read that again. If you have hope, then you will believe in your destination. Without a destination that you believe in, there is no point in even having a roadmap. So realize that there IS hope, be hopeful, have hope...and create a customized route to improve your quality of life with this book. You CAN do it.

How to use this book

I did not have a book like this when I was trying to heal my TMJ. I wish I had had a "roadmap" to help guide me 20 years ago instead of learning by trial and error. I could have felt better in less time and had more confidence in the path I was on. That is what I heard time after time when speaking with other TMJ disorder patients. This is what I desire to provide for you. I hope to be able to make a positive impact on your quality of life by sharing the information contained here. In the end, though, your results depend on you taking action. No amount of reading alone will improve your TMJ health if you do not take action. You have taken action by deciding to read this book. By doing this, you have already taken your first step forward.

Something inspired you to take that action. Keep that momentum. Take the title of this book seriously and really consider it to be "*Your* ROADMAP to TMJ Health". Using a roadmap means you are going somewhere. It implies that you have a goal. It implies action and action gets results. Where are you going? Toward TMJ health! You will define what that means to you in order to set your goals later in Section 4. Enlist the sense of action that the title implies to help you implement your plan of action that we will help you create in Section 4. You may find yourself reading the book all the way through first without taking any action and that's okay. You may want to read through it all one time and then go back and use it to make a plan of action for yourself. That's actually a great idea. Or you may take action along the way as you read. Just know that everyone is different and whatever works for you is fine as long as you are making progress toward your goal of improving your TMJ health.

Section 2: "Understanding TMJ Disorder" is dedicated to defining and understanding TMJ disorder in laypersons' words. It will assist you in identifying signs and symptoms as well as the causes and the effect of TMJ disorder on a person's quality of life. To use the roadmap analogy, think of this section as understanding the road signs.

Section 3: "Assemble Your Dream Team of Healers" will enable you to decide who will travel with you on your road to TMJ health and what vehicle you will travel in. Who will be there to support you and help you get from one point to another? Section 3 focuses on describing the treatment options, and their providers, that can be used for treating TMJ disorder. Again I will explain the treatment options in very understandable language along with their "technical" names , so that you will be prepared with the proper information when interviewing doctors and putting together your dream team of healers who will be your travel companions and co-pilots on this journey.

I have separated the chapters on treatment options by the type of medicine, therapy, or healing practiced, so that you may reference them quickly later on. You can also go straight to a specific treatment option if you really want to read about that right away. It is not necessary to have read all the portions leading up to a chapter with the exception that you should have a basic understanding on anatomy and definition of TMJ disorder. Therefore, Section 2 is recommended before reading anything else on suggested treatments and self-care.

However, this book is most beneficial if read at least once in its entirety from start to finish since, as the title suggests, it is a "roadmap" and designed to help guide you step by step through the process. You may then refer back to it when you are ready to take action on your road to TMJ health. With that in mind, treatment categories are divided by approach and then by methods within each approach.

The treatment options can be viewed as vehicles on the road to TMJ health. Here, it is useful to define where you are and where you desire to go in order to choose the best vehicle. If you were going down a bumpy dirt road, you wouldn't choose a sports car to travel there. Which leads to Section 4.

Section 4: "Destination TMJ Health" guides you in creating your roadmap to TMJ health. This section will help you to define clear and specific goals for your TMJ health since it is important to know your exact destination. Self-assessment to evaluate where you are starting from is also important. You will need to know where point A and point B are in order to know who would best help you get there. Identifying those waypoints, or goals, is covered in Section 4. You have to know where you are going in order to get there. This section will help you set goals for your TMJ health and create a plan to achieve them.

Finally, we suggest some measures you can take to create a supportive environment that is conducive to healing. After all, healing doesn't only happen in a treatment room or doctor's office. Shifting your lifestyle to one that embraces health does not mean you have to suddenly make drastic changes to your way of life. (Although you may choose to do that if that is what makes you feel supported in your health.) If living a healthy life makes you think of some stereotypical "health nut," then you are putting labels on health. For some people, the image of being a vegan who bikes to work and wears earth friendly sandals is empowering to their identity of health. It may not be for you and guess what? That is perfectly fine! If you label health as something you don't identify with, then you will not have the desire to achieve it. Forget whatever preconceived notions you have about what a "healthy lifestyle" means. If you think of ideal health in terms of an unattainable standard of perfection, you are setting yourself up for failure and disappointment. The lifestyle changes I am referring to are ways to be the best YOU in order to support your healing path at home and in your life in general. After all, your TMJ does not exist in isolation. It is part of your body as a whole and your body is both impacted by and a reflection of your life. You have the power to make choices in your life. The first step is awareness of that fact and the desire for change, the desire for health. Next comes seeking and gaining information, educating yourself and, finally, taking action.

Section 2

Understanding TMJ Disorder

Basic Anatomy of the Human Jaw

Temporomandibular Joint Disc

Joint dysfunction and pain arises when the disc is displaced either to the front, back, or side of the condyle.

Repeated displacement or direct trauma due to injury can damage the disc leaving little to no cushion between the bones of the joint

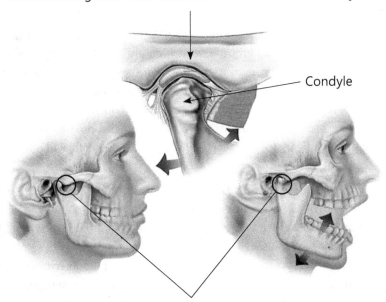

Condyle

The joint rotates and slides forward upon opening

Temporomandibular Joint (TMJ)

What is TMJ Disorder?

People who say they "have TMJ" are usually leaving off an important additional letter. The letter "D" that stands for "disorder" or "dysfunction". Saying you "have TMJ" is like saying you "have a leg". So, let's break it down letter by letter. T is for temporo, M is for mandibular, J is for joint. TMJ is simply an abbreviation for the jaw joint, healthy or unhealthy. There is one temporomandibular joint on each side of your head connecting your lower jaw to your skull. It is unique in that it is the only bi-hinge joint in your body. It is also the most used joint in your body. The unhealthy function of the joint is sometimes abbreviated as TMD, Temporo Mandibular Disorder/ Dysfunction. Additionally, the condition is sometimes abbreviated as a combination of the first two as TMJD. These are all different names for the same problem. That is, the less than ideal function of the jaw joint resulting in pain, inflammation, and possible joint deterioration.

The National Institute of Health estimates that over 10 million Americans suffer from TMJD. Additionally, The National Institute of Dental and Craniofacial Research has found that women are affected more than twice as much as men. There are even emerging studies linking estrogen levels with TMJD. This may be why younger people especially women, and women taking supplemental estrogen including contraceptives, are more affected than older people. As of the writing of this book, the reason for the hormonal link is unknown. Hopefully, more research will shed light on this aspect.

The collection of symptoms associated with TMJ disorder is also referred to as TMJ syndrome. Again, there is no difference between them. The names do not distinguish between varying levels of pain or number of symptoms. However, levels of pain as well as location of pain and number of symptoms can vary from person to person and even for one person over a period of time. It is not always immediately apparent that the symptoms are related to the jaw. This is one of the confusing and misunderstood aspects of TMJ disorder. Perhaps you are even reading this book to determine if you have TMJ disorder. Possibly, you may even help someone you know to identify TMJD related pain and therefore a potential solution. This book is not meant to be an in-depth description of TMJD itself. There are other books that go into greater detail as to the function and anatomy behind TMJD and associated symptoms. This book is meant to be a practical guide to healing by gathering, organizing and applying information to build a team of healers and healing practices that support your goals for wellness. I imagine most readers are somewhat familiar with their condition. If not, check the resources section for other sources of information on the topic. That being said, let's look at the signs and symptoms to help you identify TMJ disorder.

Signs and Symptoms

People who live with TMJ disorder may experience all, a few, or just one of the following symptoms. The symptoms may be chronic, lasting for very long periods of time, or acute, coming and going for short periods of time. Acute symptoms are usually brought on by a recent action, behavior, or change in habits. They are sometimes seasonal and, as previously mentioned, there are emerging theories on a hormonal link. Possibly, this is why most TMJD patients are female. More explanation on the reasons for chronic versus acute symptoms are discussed further in the chapter on causes below.

• Pain/aching/soreness in the actual jaw joint

This may be felt as throbbing pain, or aching dull pain, or a sharp pain upon opening and/or closing depending on the condition of the structures of the joint.

• Pain/aching/soreness of the associated muscles/tendons of the joint

This may be felt as tenderness and/or stiffness/tightness in any of the muscles and tendons of the face/jaw/neck. Sometimes felt as muscle spasms, twitching, and or tingling. Can sometimes be seen as "knots" or swelling due to inflammation.

• Pain in the neck and shoulders; can be either sharp stabbing pain or a dull aching or both.

Stiffness and tightness in the neck and shoulders can impact the TMJ and vice-versa. Poor posture of the head, neck, and back can not only cause strain and misalignment of those areas, but also of the TMJ. On the other hand, having TMJD can lead to unhealthy posture due to the pain and dysfunction of the jaw. It's one of those "chicken or the egg" things; which one comes first? Hard to say unless you have a very specific situation like you had no TMJ problems and then got into a car accident, had whiplash, and the damage to your neck led to TMJD.

- pain/aching/soreness in the face, possibly extending to the scalp

Can feel like a generalized headache or as hypersensitivity on the skin like a bruise or a "pins and needles" tingling sensation.

- pain/aching/soreness in the ear and ringing in the ear (tinnitus). Popping, crackling, or crunching sounds in the ear are also very common.
- Clicking, popping, or grinding sounds that people in close proximity can hear when opening and closing the mouth.

Can sound like "cracking knuckles," or like sandpaper, or a variety of sounds from hardly noticeable to very noticeable. The sounds are caused by either the position of the cartilage and the bone popping on and off the cartilage, or by the bone rubbing on bone or by tight connective tissue rubbing against another structure (muscle, tendon, ligament or bone).

- Difficulty chewing

This can be experienced with every bite or just occasionally while chewing. It may be impossible to chew hard foods without experiencing extreme pain or locking up of the joint. It may also be experienced as fatigue with the progression of a meal to the point where the jaw feels too tired to chew anymore. Chewing can feel exhausting and the jaw becomes weaker and more dysfunctional with every bite. Often manual assistance is needed by easing the jaw into position with one's hand and a rubbing/massaging action on the outside of the face.

- Difficulty opening and/or closing the mouth

Similar to chewing, the same symptoms may occur during speaking or any other activity that requires opening and closing of the mouth.

- Locking of the jaw in open or closed position

The jaw muscles may get fatigued and "lock up" the joint in a disoriented position. Another "stuck" sensation may happen when the cartilage disk is displaced either in front of or behind its normal position.

- Abnormal wear on teeth

Clenching or grinding of the teeth can happen during the day or at night while sleeping. Clenching/grinding, referred to as "bruxism," can cause TMJD, or it can be a symptom of TMJD. Either way, the force to the teeth can cause damage by wearing down enamel, causing cracks and fractures, and/or stressing the nerve to the point of needing a root canal.

- Tooth pain

When nerves of the jaw and face are inflamed, they can cause referred pain. The nerves that connect to the teeth can express painful sensations that feel like a toothache even though the teeth themselves may be completely healthy. Or the teeth may be damaged by abnormal wear and are painful due to that damage.

- Headaches

Can be mild to very severe, even mistaken for migraines. Sensitivity to light and sound can occur. May be in combination with stabbing/shooting pain behind eye and/or ear on the same side as the affected joint.

- Sleep apnea

The unhealthy position of the dysfunctional jaw can restrict the airway causing disrupted sleep. The relationship of TMJD and sleep apnea is only recently becoming more widely understood. Furthermore, devices to treat sleep apnea can affect the jaw joint, so it is important to take TMJD into consideration when treating sleep apnea.

Causes

Now let's delve into the question why. Why is there dysfunction in the jaw and what causes it? It is only by addressing the cause and not just treating the symptoms that true healing can begin. Treating symptoms may result in temporary relief and while that is helpful until the more long-term plan can be laid out, it is not a good strategy for success later on down the road. There are different causes for this disorder and there may be overlap between them.

Some people are born with structures not correctly formed. A person can have an anatomical abnormality that affects the function and health of the TMJ. Misshaped structures of the TMJ can be either in the hard tissue like bone or soft tissue like tendons. Also, there is a genetic component to the breakdown in these structures even if they were formed correctly at birth. Some people may have been born with healthy jaw joint discs that for some reason are prone to deteriorate and cause arthritis later on. Just like having "bad knees" runs in families, so too can TMJD. Having a "bad bite", known as severe malocclusion, can definitely cause TMJD and is usually something you are born with. The lower jaw can grow farther than the upper jaw or shorter than the upper jaw causing all of the teeth to be out of alignment. This is one of the reasons for having braces especially at a young age when the jaw is still developing. Finally, any systemic inflammatory disease that has a genetic component could also contribute to TMJD. Conditions like rheumatoid arthritis, fibromyalgia, and neuralgia can mimic TMJD like symptoms, even if the jaw joint is not structurally dysfunctional, but they can also be present along with TMJD.

Speaking of conditions present along with TMJD, it is worth mentioning here that there is a relationship in medicine with the awful name of co-morbidity. Co-morbidity is another name for associated or co-existing conditions. There are certain conditions that are present along with TMJD, but the cause and effect relationship is not clearly understood. What this means is that the occurrence of these other conditions in people with TMJD is noted so often that it is not simply coincidence. Studies by the National Institute of Health report that these conditions are up to six times more likely in TMJD patients. Some common other co-existing conditions to be aware of (in addition to fibromyalgia and arthritis) are migraines, chronic fatigue syndrome, sleep apnea, irritable bowel syndrome, allergies, depression and restless leg syndrome. There has been some research recently that seems to support that the longer someone has TMJD and the higher the pain levels are, the greater the chances are that they will have more of the associated conditions. This is something to consider when seeking treatment and is another reason why a comprehensive approach is so important.

Injury or trauma is another cause of TMJD that might sound obvious, but can sometimes be difficult to identify as a cause. Car accidents, whiplash, a violent assault, such as a punch in the face, or a sports injury can damage the TMJ. However, many times after healing from the initial trauma, people don't realize that the TMJ is still damaged especially if treatment was never aimed at healing the jaw joint and related structures, especially if there were more severe injuries that took the attention away from the TMJ. The effect of the injury on the TMJ may not be recognized until much later. By the time the TMJ disorder is detected, it may be hard to connect the dots as to the injury or trauma that caused it.

There is a cause of TMJD that comes from treatment received by a doctor called iatrogenic. It does not mean that a doctor necessarily did something wrong as in malpractice. It could be that a procedure or treatment you had resulted in the unwanted side effect of stress or damage to the TMJ. For example, someone having their wisdom teeth extracted might experience TMJ problems after the surgery due to the position of the jaw and length of time in that position during the surgery. Orthodontics, either by braces or by aligners, can cause TMJ problems. Even though it is also a treatment to correct the bite, it can in some cases make matters worse. It depends on why the orthodontic treatment is being done and what the actual results are as to how the patient's teeth and jaw respond to the treatment. What was the goal of the orthodontic treatment and was it successful? Just because the teeth are straight does not mean the bite is balanced and what was the relationship of the jaw joint before during and after treatment? This can all be monitored with imaging. Seemingly simple dental work can also have a lasting effect on the TMJ. A filling, crown, or anything that can impact the way your teeth touch together has the potential to aggravate the TMJ and lead to pretty severe discomfort. Again, like the injury scenario, it may not be immediately apparent that the dental work caused the TMJ problem. Especially if it is a very small discrepancy, it may take years of chronic imbalance to stress the TMJ to the point where it flares up.

Dino has had several cases where his patient was having pretty severe TMJ pain that was resolved with a simple occlusal adjustment. In these cases, previous dental work was done that created a small change in the person's bite; once corrected, no other treatment for TMJ pain was needed.

Certain habits, and these can be conscious or unconscious, can cause so much stress to the TMJ that it causes TMJD. Chronic stressors like chewing gum, ice, fingernails, and objects like pens all put regular added stress on the jaw joint and related structures. Opening packages, bottles or containers with teeth are habits that can damage the TMJ. Bruxism (clenching and/or grinding teeth) is a major cause of TMJD. Some people grind their teeth only at night, other people clench throughout the day, some clench and/or grind day and night. Just imagine the stress this puts on the TMJ and all the muscles of the neck and jaw! Many people don't even realize they are doing it, but the evidence is in their teeth as they wear down and even break their teeth due to the severe strain. Believe it or not, some people are in denial that they grind and/or clench their teeth because they either do it only at night, or they are so unaware of themselves that they don't realize they are doing it.

As previously mentioned, there is a possible hormone link with the very high percentage of women afflicted. Approximately 90% of TMJD patients are women of childbearing age. It may be physiological/hormonal; however, I personally have my own theory that it is at least partially stress related. Women of childbearing age often are balancing work and family with small children. They are very emotional beings who feel responsible for caring for their family and put a lot of pressure on themselves. Their family, especially their children, depend on them for everyday needs. Even if they are not the ones performing the tasks personally, they are still the CEO of the household and the ones usually managing, coordinating, and supervising to be sure everyone's needs are met. This is a lot of responsibility. This brings us to the next cause and one that is very important. Even if other causes are identified, this next one should never be ignored.

Mental health and emotional well-being cannot be overlooked. This non-physical perspective impacts every part of our physical being. First, I want to stress that non-physical does not mean that the problem is not real. I am a firm believer that physical illness, pain, and dysfunction is our body's way of communicating to us about our life choices. However, the pain does exist and the dysfunction is real. It can be infuriating for someone in pain to hear another person blow off their suffering by saying, "it's all in your head". And if anyone has ever said something like this to you, it may predispose you to being close minded and defensive toward the mental/ emotional/spiritual side of healing. I urge you to let the past go and look at this information with fresh eyes. Your ability to heal will be tremendously impacted by your attitude about this. Disorder and dysfunction essentially mean that things are not "in-order" and not functioning properly. When aspects of your life are not in order and not functioning in a healthy way, it can show up as one or many physical manifestations in your body.

Stress shows itself in many ways in our bodies. One place it can and often does show up is in the neck, shoulders, head, and jaw. The TMJ is a dynamic joint influenced by posture. Tension in the neck and shoulders and/or poor postural habits can affect the TMJ. In my interview with Dr. Anthony B. Morovati, a chiropractor with extensive experience in pain management including TMJD, he says that in his experience about 80-85% of TMJD is soft tissue in origin. Meaning that the cause is not a joint that needs surgery or other invasive treatment. In the majority of cases he has seen over his 30 plus years of practice, successful treatment was based on soft tissue management and a collaborative approach among healthcare providers. This should be a source of hope because achieving healthy soft tissue to support healthy joint function is relatively inexpensive compared to addressing other causes. Every person's body holds stress in different ways according to their habits, the way their body is built, and where they are vulnerable due to injury or illness. Monitoring your stress level in your Wellness Journal is one way to see how and where your body responds to stress.

Effect on Quality of Life

Are you aware of how living with TMJ disorder is impacting your quality of life? You may be very aware and have no problem detailing exactly how TMJD is affecting your life. I was not aware until my TMJ dysfunction became quite severe and caused me a good amount of pain. What I remember most, though, is the aching that was a constant distraction that kept me from focusing. Some people with TMJD have expressed not wanting to eat in the company of others due to embarrassment of the clicking and popping noises their jaw makes. I have heard from some with TMJD that they are self-conscious about their appearance because their smile is not symmetrical or their jaw is swollen or more heavily muscled on one side vs the other. I have heard too many people with TMJD express suicidal thoughts from the feeling of hopelessness combined with pain. You may not experience very bad pain or discomfort, but the jaw dysfunction may still have a negative impact on your health and/or quality of life.

Next let's evaluate how the symptoms of TMJ disorder can affect someone's quality of life. You can use these as prompts to help you with Worksheet 2 – "Quality of Life Goals" later in Section 4.

- Do you suffer from distracting aches and pains associated with your jaw? This can impact your interaction with people in the workplace, as well as friends and family. When you are not present, people notice even if they don't say anything. The funny thing is, people usually take it personally thinking it is something about them you don't like. To take it a step further, if you are having a bad flare-up and are experiencing pain, you may take it out on those around you without meaning to. You may find yourself short tempered, grouchy, grumpy, irritable, and downright angry. How do you think that is affecting your relationships with your children, spouse, friends, and co-workers?

- Do you avoid speaking in public? Jaw pain and dysfunction could be one reason you don't like to speak up in meetings or social groups. Also, if you are self-conscious about your appearance like some people with TMJD, it may undermine your confidence even if you are not having pain.

- Are you a performer? Singing, acting, and dancing on stage could all be impacted by TMJD. Prolonged periods of singing and speaking would be a challenge for those with TMJD. Musicians who use their mouth, head, and neck to play an instrument are also at risk of poor performance from TMJD. Some people who may love to participate in these activities are discouraged from doing so because of TMJD.

- Speaking to people all day causes extreme pain and/or jaw fatigue. Even if you are not performing on stage, TMJD symptoms could be holding you back in life. Many occupations require long hours on the phone speaking to people. It would be hard to excel in a field where you are expected to speak all day if speaking aggravates your TMJD.

- Difficulty enjoying a meal. As mentioned above, this could be either from not being able to physically chew properly, pain related to chewing, or being self-conscious about jaw sounds and appearance while eating. This impacts quality of life in two ways. One, nutritionally as in you may not be getting all the nutrients you need due to food avoidance. When implementing a soft-foods diet, it is important to include nutritional ingredients. Second, eating is social. This actually impacts relationships in and out of the workplace. Many family gatherings and workplace meetings and events are held around meals. Are you excluding yourself from these occasions because of your TMJD symptoms?

- Unable to enjoy sexual intimacy. Many people with TMJD report not being able to tolerate even the gentlest caress of the face or head. Kissing may also be a challenge or very uncomfortable if not seemingly impossible. Oral sex may be literally non-existent. All of this is not helpful in having a fully satisfying intimate relationship.

- Are you unable to get a good night's sleep? TMJD often interrupts sleep patterns and is one of the causes of sleep apnea. Restful and restorative sleep is essential for overall wellness. Lack of sleep contributes to serious health problems like heart disease, high blood pressure, and diabetes. Not to mention how terrible it makes you feel being groggy, not able to concentrate, performing poorly on the job, or possibly falling asleep at the wheel.

Section 3

Assemble Your Dream Team!

A team approach to
TMJ health and putting together
your team of healers

Why You Need a Team of Healers.

"Teamwork divides the task and multiplies the success"

~ Unknown

"Sometimes the most ordinary things could be made extraordinary simply by doing them with the right people"

~ Nicholas Sparks

Why do you need a team? This was touched on in Section 1 regarding why a roadmap is beneficial. Here we talk more about the importance of a comprehensive approach to TMJ health. One of the biggest obstacles we have seen preventing people from getting lasting relief from TMJ related pain is that they get treatment from one doctor/practitioner or another at a time and rarely coordinate treatment methods from different disciplines. Some fortunate individuals are guided by open-minded healers who know that a comprehensive approach is the way to go for successful lasting results. If you are one of these people, count yourself very lucky! A health-care provider who truly cares about the best interest of their patient is the one who embraces all options that can potentially help their patient. There are some people who are very involved in taking responsibility for their healthcare and may seek out every option available and research it to figure out if they should try it. Those individuals may also have luck with their results, although they may experience some trial and error along the way. For example, one of the TMJ patients I interviewed eventually took her health and quality of life in her own hands by coordinating Eastern medicine (energetic healing and acupuncture) with Western medicine "(orthodontics and surgery) along with chiropractic care to get the results she was looking for. However, it took her a good portion of her life to reach that point since she carved out that path on her own. Had she known earlier what is presented here in this book, she could have avoided several traumatic experiences and improved her quality of life sooner. Another interview subject revealed to me that she wished she had known earlier how helpful therapy for a traumatic physical and emotional issue would be for her TMJD. She first treated it with some success by an appliance made by her dentist. However, it was only after addressing an underlying past trauma that she had the greatest relief.

Every doctor I interviewed who has had success treating TMJD patients stressed the importance of a team approach. An approach that views the TMJ as a part of the entire person as a whole and not just a joint in isolation has the greatest results. The University of Southern California Center for Orofacial Pain & Oral Medicine teaches a course for dentists that my husband, Dr. Dino Bonyadi, has attended that also calls for a multidisciplinary approach. The program advises collecting a very thorough health history in order to examine the disorder and its relationship to the person as a whole. That being said, let's look at the signs and symptoms to help you identify TMJ disorder.

A comprehensive multidisciplinary approach to healing can be applied to any health problem to achieve the best possible results. However, the many causes and effects of TMJD demand that it is addressed comprehensively. In a way, the fact that there is not one standardized accepted and designated "TMJ specialist" can be looked at as a positive thing. It forces us to look at the entire body and not just the jaw. The jaw does not exist in isolation. It is part of your whole body and it is connected with nerves and muscles and tendons and other structures. Treating only the teeth, or only the bones, or only the muscles, etc., is not solving the problem because TMJD is a collection of varying symptoms from the imbalance in various structures. Even if there is one sole cause of your TMJD, the effect of the disorder on other structures and your overall health should be addressed. Finding solutions to the main cause is important, of course, but the chronic strain and/or damage to other structures can become problems in and of themselves and continue to cause pain and discomfort even after the main cause of your TMJD is resolved. And, as previously discussed, the affected structures can be different from person to person. This is what leads to the frustration and confusion so heartbreaking and prevalent among TMJD patients. It is also why a customized healing plan designed for your specific situation is important to get the best results for improving your quality of life.

So rather than trial and error and jumping from one doctor or health-care provider to another, we will help you create a thoughtful plan that includes your dream team of healers. Now this team can be different for everyone and does not need to include every type of practitioner below. It is most important that the healthcare providers support each other's treatment modes and value what each brings to the table. That brings us to the first requirement for your dream team: an open-minded attitude toward therapies that are not provided by them. This can mean therapies not actually performed by them or therapies that are outside their area of expertise. Some doctors and other healthcare providers are reluctant to accept that anything but what they do can help you. There is no one cure-all for any medical problem, so this narrow-minded attitude has no place in healing people or improving people's lives by reducing pain. Dino experienced this first-hand as a patient himself when he was suffering greatly with pain from cluster headaches. When I say pain, I mean drop-you-to-the-floor, suicidal pain. He sought help from a trusted physician who prescribed him drugs with side-effects not acceptable to Dino and told him he just had to live with it. A neurologist also prescribed drugs and told him there was nothing else that could help him. A short while later, Dino experienced relief thanks to Dr. Anthony B. Morovati, a chiro-practor who utilized several treatment methods in addition to adjustment (micro-current technology, acupressure, and others). This along with some lifestyle changes allowed him to avoid prescription drugs and have his life back. This is because his chiropractor looked at his headaches as part of the whole body. He asked the important question, "what is going on in the rest of the body and why? What is going on in the person's life?" The trusted physician he first visited later scoffed at him in arrogance when Dino told him that a chiropractor had healed his cluster headaches. If my husband had simply handed over his health to the first doctor, there is no telling what amount of suffering he would have continued to endure and where that would have led. I am sure it would have been a very dark road. It is this kind of experience we wish to help you avoid.

In order to help you to select members of your dream team, we have provided sample interview questions for your "interviews". Yes, interviews. Did you ever realize when you go to a doctor or other healthcare provider that you are not just there to be examined? That you should be actively engaged and looking for certain traits in your practitioner? How do you find these traits? If they are not openly advertised, then you will find out by asking questions. When you research and then call a healthcare provider you can conduct part of the interview to see if you should even move on to "part 2". Part 2 can be conducted during the initial exam or consultation.

(Please see the Workbook at the back of the book
for the sample interview questions.)

Where to Begin

Your first step on the road to TMJ health begins with you.

"Open your eyes, look within.
Are you satisfied with the life you're living?"

~ Bob Marley

"Knowing yourself is the beginning of all wisdom."

~ Aristotle

Before you look outside yourself to assemble your team, let's make sure you are on your team. The first step of any journey is to evaluate where you are at a given moment in time. By reading this book, you have put at least one foot on the road to a healthy pain free TMJ. In order to get to that destination, you need to take a look around at yourself and your life before you take the next step. In order to get your bearings, you will ask yourself some questions and be willing to listen to the answer. Ask yourself the following questions:

1. Am I willing to take responsibility for my health?

This is a big one and may seem like a simple or strange question to some. There are people who want to hand over all their power to a doctor to "just make them better". They don't want to think about or play an active role in the decision making process regarding treatment options. Many people want their doctor to prescribe them a "magic pill" to make their problem go away rather than take a proactive role by being informed and accepting responsibility for their own bodies. For example, just look at the prescription drug epidemic in the United States. Another challenge to overcoming any health issue is having a "victim mind-set". Do you blame others for all of your problems? Is there someone or something that you blame for your TMJD? If so then you might be taking on the role of a victim and by doing so you hand over all of your power to those that you blame. If you have had that attitude in the past or maybe still do, please realize that you must be the steward of your body and your health. While you will seek help from trusted healthcare practitioners, you must be actively involved in the process and not just a passenger on this journey. It is in your own best interest to be in the driver's seat on your journey to health. This is important both in the process of building your team and during the active treatment phase. During the selection process, you should listen to your instincts when deciding if a practitioner is the right match for you. You both must be on the same page if you are to collaborate as partners for your benefit. This is a bit of a balancing act because while you maintain ultimate responsibility for your life and your health, you must also have a certain level of trust in your healthcare providers. When you have found practitioners you can trust, you must be willing and able to listen to and understand their recommendations no matter how difficult it may be. They may need to tell you something you don't want to hear and/or you may feel overwhelmed by your situation. When you take responsibility for the decision making regarding your healthcare choices, it can be overwhelming if it is a new experience for you. Take a breath, keep an open mind, and ask questions. Don't automatically resist an idea or course of treatment as soon as it is presented to you. Take your time to find out more about it and try not to pass judgement on the treatment, the practitioner, or yourself. Educate yourself in order to make the best decisions. Don't just do something because someone tells you to. Ask questions and listen to the answers. Do not "react;" think and then respond with the appropriate action.

Too often we see people who are currently answering "no" to question number 1. For example, when Dino was consulting with a patient whose damage to her teeth was a sign of the likely cause of her almost constant headaches, he brought it to her attention. She was clenching her jaw and grinding her teeth down to the point that many of them would soon need restorative dental work in order to retain their basic function. She was a tense ball of stress and she brushed it off saying she would take care of herself when this, that, or the other thing was done and she had more time. She was obviously putting everyone and everything else in her life first and her general health had also deteriorated. She was not ready to accept that if she didn't make her health a priority, nobody else would. Therefore, her teeth and jaw will continue to suffer and her TMJ related problems worsen until something motivates her to change. It may take a broken tooth or severe jaw, head, and neck pain to be a wake up call and spur her into action. This is actually an all too common scenario. And one that can be prevented. You can choose health. It's up to you to decide.

A little different scenario is that of one of my interview subjects. Ann lived with a fairly severe case of TMJ disorder and attempted to seek treatment for it several times over a period of 40 years. Each time she went to a different doctor and had a few traumatic experiences. Early in her life, when she was young woman in her 20s, a dentist advised her to extract all her teeth and make dentures. Yes, as a solution to her jaw problem, a doctor advised her to pull out all of her healthy teeth. She was young and trusting and this was 1968, so she even went ahead with the first appointment. Fortunately, her instincts kicked in and she did not continue down that path. However, she was severely scarred by the experience. It undermined her trust in doctors and prevented her from following through on her initial plan for wellness. Eventually, over ten years later, she ventured out on the path again. She underwent lengthy orthodontic treatment wearing metal braces with wires as an adult to correct misaligned teeth. But lacking a comprehensive approach, this was not enough to resolve her TMJD and perhaps could have made it worse. Only her misaligned teeth were addressed, nothing else. In any case, she did not wear retainers and her teeth migrated back to their pre-braces position. Another 20 plus years went by before Ann attempted to get back on the road to TMJ health. It was after experiencing her worst symptoms that included sharp pain into her ears and not being able to eat due to the pain and position of her jaw. Her jaw felt disoriented and she would have to go through a series of maneuvers in order to open and close her mouth. Ann finally decided to seek out a team who could help her. She did not consciously set out to have a team. It was in large part due to how much she had grown as a person with regard to her perspectives about life and her approach to health and wellness in general that influenced this next phase of her journey. Her personal development led her to have a healthier and more aware approach around achieving her desire of a functional and healthy TMJ. She took responsibility by educating herself and doing research on TMJD and treatment options available to her within a reasonable distance. She also incorporated visualization and positive mind-set into her healing. She became the driver on her road to TMJ health. She made a conscious decision to do everything in her power to have the best outcome that she could imagine. Her research led her to find a team of doctors she trusted. Ann had orthodontic treatment again (two years in braces) and then underwent jaw surgery to correct the misalignment of her lower jaw to her upper jaw and at the time was her surgeon's most extreme case of repositioning. During her ortho treatment and recovery from surgery, she practiced gratitude and visualizing her doctors telling her that she was the most successful case they have had. Her mind-set was so strong, she even recovered from surgery without prescription painkillers. She was willing and committed to do whatever she could to support her health including researching, informing herself, and seeking treatment from supportive therapies like chiropractic, acupuncture, and energetic healing as well as being diligent about self-care. As a result, Ann is in the healthiest state she has been in her life and she hasn't stopped seeking out wellness.

The good news is, you can always choose to say "yes" to this question! Even if you haven't in the past. You can start now. In Section 4 we include a secret weapon to help you stay committed to this path. It's the "Wellness Pledge" and it is a simple but powerful tool.

2- Do I listen to my body?

If you are not already in touch with your body, learn to listen to it. Your body is giving you feedback all the time. Think of pain as a sign, part of a language for your body to communicate with you to help you care for it better. To raise your level of awareness about your body regarding TMJ pain and dysfunction, consider keeping a diary or journal. Make notes with dated entries regarding your pain level, location of pain, type of pain, clicking, or other dysfunction. Be as descriptive as possible. You don't need to have information going back years, but any period of time you can keep track of will not only help you be more aware of your body , but also help your healing team to better help you. (We have included a Wellness Journal in the Workbook as a starting point for you.)

If you are interested in deepening your body awareness, the following activities can be tried. Mindful breathing & meditation is where you still your mind and focus your attention inward. If you are not familiar with these techniques or have a hard time doing this in the beginning, you can find guided meditation downloads online. Physical practices that improve body awareness include yoga, tai chi, and Feldenkrais. Practices like these focus on achieving harmony and balance in your physical being that also overflows into other areas of your life. Being more aware of your body will allow you to catch the signs and signals your body gives before experiencing full on pain, dysfunction, and deterioration. Learning your body's early warning signs is an invaluable tool for prevention.

3. Am I in an acute flare-up and needing immediate relief? Or am I in a chronic pain cycle?

Again this is where keeping track with a journal will help. For acute pain and dysfunction, take note of activities you engaged in just prior to the onset. This, of course, includes foods you ate, giving long talks, dental appointments, and all those activities you directly use your mouth and jaw for. However, don't omit other activities or events going on in your personal life. Did you argue with your spouse or child? Did something change at work? Make note of any recent changes in your daily life. It doesn't need to be a novel. It is up to you how much you want to document. Be sure, though, to include the important facts like the severity of the pain and detail when and where the pain or dysfunction occurs.

For more chronic conditions, it may be a bit more challenging. This is because you may have become accustomed to living with a certain amount of pain and/or dysfunction. It has become normal for you. In this case, documentation is a little more like detective work. You will begin to look for clues and see where that leads. Try to think of things you avoid doing because of your TMJD and when the last time you can remember doing them was.

Finally, ask yourself the following two part question.

4. What have I done or tried already? Has it helped?

Make a list of things you have done, doctors you have seen, treatments you have tried, and what the results were from each. Also note when they were done.

Who are potential team members?

Team members are people you will place in your Circle of Wellness and could include any or all of the following practitioners, but remember it begins with you!

Will you need to have a member from each of the categories below on your team? No, not necessarily. Please do not look at this section in its entirety and let it overwhelm you. The entire point of this book is to help you take it step by step, one day at a time. There is some overlap regarding approach and type of treatment between doctors and other healers. You may find that some are a part of your team short term and others more long term. You could, over time, have all of them included in your Circle of Wellness at one point or another and not necessarily all at the same time. I have attempted to be as comprehensive as possible in order for you to have more options to choose from depending on what is available to you in your part of the world. During the interviews I conducted with different health-care providers, the valuable point I took away was that it is most important for your practitioners to value the input of the entire team and not to be "lone rangers".

To use the roadmap analogy, think of each treatment option again as the vehicle for a certain portion of the route along the way on your road to TMJ health. Some sections of the road will be shorter than others, but each will allow you to move forward to the next stop. However, resist the temptation to think of the road as a straight line. This is not a linear journey. (See "Circle of Wellness" diagram also available as a digital download.) Set yourself up for success by being willing to accept where each phase of treatment takes you and then moving on from there. Remember when I said you could change course or revise your roadmap?

(To help summarize these options and integrate them with
the information you compiled on yourself, we have included a
"Roadmap Builder" tool. It can be found in the
workbook section of the book and also as a free download.)

So now let's take a look at the different options for doctors and other healthcare practitioners as well as the treatments provided by each. This list is not meant to be exclusive. Please feel free to include any practitioners you feel would contribute to your "Circle of Wellness". This is YOUR dream team and you can include whomever you desire. This list is a good starting point to build a foundation for you to expand on if you want to.

MD or other type of Family Physician

- Your primary care doctor may be a first point of contact for diagnosing TMJD signs and symptoms and should definitely be included due to the high occurrence of co-existing conditions. A general practitioner should rule out or rule in any other underlying causes such as systemic inflammatory diseases or other conditions that may seem like TMJD (having similar symptoms). Also, remember that it is common for people with TMJD to have a coinciding ailment. The connection is not exactly known for all the related diseases, but the following co-existing conditions (also referred to as co-morbidity) that often appear along with TMJD should be addressed. Other conditions that often occur along with TMJD are allergies, depression, chronic fatigue syndrome, degenerative arthritis, fibromyalgia, auto-immune disorders, sleep apnea, and gastrointestinal problems like irritable bowel syndrome and gluten intolerance. A systemic inflammatory condition may not be the primary cause of your TMJD, but it will surely have a negative effect on it. This is why it is important to approach TMJD comprehensively, not just looking at the jaw joint, but taking into consideration the person and their entire body as a whole. Your doctor may recommend medications to help with pain and inflammation from TMJD. Prescription and over the counter medications should be taken into consideration by weighing the pros and cons of taking them. Take note and discuss with your doctor the following questions: Are you taking any now? Is it for another condition? How does it affect the TMJ? For example, there are prescription antidepressants that have a known side effect of causing clenching. So even if you don't think it's related, ask. If you are prescribed anything as a result of seeking treatment for TMJD, ask how it may interact with any other medications you are taking. Also, it's always a good idea to educate yourself on any medications you are taking that have been prescribed for you. Your primary care doctor may refer you to an appropriate specialist for any systemic condition that is identified. While they address and treat any conditions that may coincide with TMJD, your doctor may also refer you to a knowledgeable/trusted dentist, chiropractor, and/or other practitioner type mentioned below. If they don't offer, you can ask for a referral.

Dentist

- TMJD can be discovered or diagnosed during routine dental checkups. Dentistry is not limited to only the structures inside of the mouth. A thorough head and neck exam including the TMJ should be part of your general dentist's regular exam. A thorough exam should include all of these areas as well as inside the mouth such as teeth and gums. Once TMJD is suspected, a more thorough evaluation of not only the jaw, but of your health history will likely be needed for further diagnosis. This may mean additional x-rays and other imaging and a more specific TMJD related exam to determine the type and degree of dysfunction. The following are some less invasive dental options for treating TMJD: Bite guards – an appliance that can be worn over the upper or lower teeth. Usually worn on top to avoid constricting the tongue. The general purpose is to get a balanced bite, known as occlusion. This is to help place the jaw in a chosen position that is less stressful and healthier for the joint. Another purpose of bite guards is to soften the impact on the teeth and protect the teeth from clenching and grinding forces. Basically, to be a protective cushion between the upper and lower teeth. The third purpose is to deprogram facial muscles. Muscles have memory. The muscles of the jaw and face may be in spasm and/or have been trained to function improperly in order to adapt to the dysfunction in the jaw. There are several names for bite guards such as occlusal guard, night guard, and orthotic. Some names refer to a specific "brand". They are all types of the same appliance. Some focus more on balancing the bite, some focus more on deprogramming, others serve only to protect the teeth. There are even hybrids combining those. Bite guards can be made of material varying in hardness and thickness depending on their purpose. One that has been very popular with Dino's patients is hard acrylic on the outside with softer material on the inside where it fits onto the teeth. This allows for patient comfort and shock absorption while still being able to adjust the outside to balance the bite. Discuss the type of bite guard your dentist recommends and ask why they recommend that type. Other potential treatments provided by your dentist could include nerve block injections, Botox injections, prescription anti-inflammatories, and muscle relaxers. One treatment that can be either very minor or very major is adjustment or correction of occlusion. When the bite is slightly off due to a small discrepancy, it can often create pretty severe TMJD symptoms. Sometimes a small adjustment is all that is needed to correct the problem and alleviate the majority of pain and discomfort. However, this should be limited to minor adjustments. If the bite is severely imbalanced and major dental work is needed to correct the problem and restore balance, then you are looking at a much more invasive approach. A bite guard to balance the bite can be made and tried before investing in the time, money, and permanent changes that extensive dental work involves. If finding the ideal position of your teeth and jaw with the bite guard produces significant improvement, you can proceed with the more permanent changes. If it does not, then you must reconsider if your bite is having an effect on your TMJD.

- Dental Specialists and why they may be involved. Depending on the cause of your TMJD, your general dentist may refer you to a specialist for further evaluation and treatment. Below is a brief overview of dental specialists and their area of expertise.

Orthodontist: Orthodontics involves moving the position of the teeth by brackets and wires or removable aligners. It is a permanent change to correct malocclusion, but the impact to the TMJ must be considered. Orthodontic treatment that results in a less than ideal outcome, or is not completed, can cause TMJD and further orthodontic treatment may be needed to correct that. Many people think that orthodontics is done to straighten the teeth only for cosmetic reasons. While this may be one reason, a very important goal is achieving a balanced bite where all the teeth come together in the most ideal way for proper function of the teeth and jaw.

Prosthodontist: May be needed in the case that many teeth need restoration and to achieve correct balance, if the general dentist is not highly skilled or experienced and/or does not have access to a dental lab that is highly skilled and experienced in attaining balance when making what is commonly referred to as "crowns" or "bridges" and other laboratory made dental restorations. As mentioned in the causes of TMJD, there is a preventive aspect to addressing these issues (iatrogenic). Keeping in mind the effect on the TMJ when having dental work done is important to prevent causing TMJD or making it much worse.

Oral Surgeon: Oral surgery needs to be ruled out right away by determining the cause of TMJD, i.e., severe malocclusion or trauma. If surgical intervention is needed, then all other treatment in the meantime will only be palliative. That is, it may help to relieve pain and discomfort, but it is not addressing the root cause. Of course, surgery is an invasive and permanent option, so a thorough evaluation and understanding of the "why" behind the surgery is of utmost importance. The risks and the benefits must be weighed according to your individual situation. Some people I interviewed had excellent results from surgery that prolonged the health of their jaw joint for years. There are several different reasons for surgery, so it is really important to find out what dysfunction a particular procedure addresses and if that is going to help you. In order to know if it is going to help you, you need to identify the type of dysfunction going on in your jaw. Finally, even if the surgical procedure is a success, that doesn't mean you can ignore all other therapies and self-care to support wellness after it is done. In other words, having surgery doesn't mean you can just go on as if you never had TMJD. Surgery is not a magic wand that will erase all of your TMJD issues. It is one potential part of your overall wellness plan for TMJ health.

Chiropractor

- Chiropractic treatment is considered in keeping with the mind-set that your TMJ does not exist in isolation. Most people are familiar with the fact that chiropractors adjust the alignment of your skeletal system. Correcting misalignments that cause stress to the soft tissue like muscles, tendons, and ligaments can help alleviate strain on the TMJ. Adjustment by a chiropractor to achieve healthy alignment of your entire body can help support your overall wellness and therefore help you be in a more balanced state to support TMJ health.

In addition to alignment, there are other therapies aimed more directly at healing a specific area of pain or discomfort. Some of these therapies may overlap with treatments provided by physical therapists or even some specially trained massage therapists. These are micro-current and shock-wave therapies that send electrical signals or sound waves to the stressed or damaged tissue. Like all treatments performed by any provider, the appropriate treatment for the cause of your discomfort is important to achieve the best results. Here again, knowing yourself and being aware of your body will help you. You should be aware or try to find out if your pain or discomfort is from injury, chronic stress, acute stress or strain, repetitive posture, or a systemic disease. Then you can evaluate whether or not a treatment presented to you will be of benefit. Ask how the treatment or therapy works and how or why it can help you.

Physical Therapist

- Generally, a physical therapist applies some therapeutic treatments for pain relief while you are visiting them and also educates you on exercises you can do at home to help rehabilitate your injured or weak area. They may have you do the exercises in their presence to train you and be sure you are doing them correctly. Exercises can and usually do include stretching and massage to aid healing and reduce pain and discomfort as well as to strengthen and condition the area to prevent future damage. They may incorporate any or all of the additional therapeutic treatments used by chiropractors with the exception of adjusting the skeletal system for alignment. Everything mentioned in the section above for chiropractic medicine about evaluating treatments and deciding if they are appropriate for your condition applies to physical therapy as well.

Acupuncturist

- It is an oversimplification to say that acupuncture is the practice of placing thin, small needles through the skin at various points to alleviate pain and promote healing. A Chinese healing tradition that dates back at least 20 centuries, acupuncture stimulates the body to heal itself by influencing energetic points and channels that exist throughout the body. In addition to treatment that would benefit TMJD specifically, acupuncture can also help support the entire immune system to help balance the body and position you for optimal wellness. This next statement is my own personal opinion; that the successful use of acupuncture is highly dependent on the practitioner. In my experience and the experience of those I have discussed this with, there seems to be an intuitiveness and "feel" that an acupuncturist has who gets great results. The same can be said for any of the healing arts that use hands-on techniques. This goes for massage therapists and chiropractors as well as dentists and surgeons. Acupressure operates on the same theory as acupuncture, only pressure is used instead of needles.

It is worth mentioning here a device that I like to refer to as "acupuncture on steroids". It's called an acuscope or equiscope (it is also used to treat horses) or myopulse machine, depending on the model. Different models are used to treat different types of injury or dysfunction in the body, but all use electrical currents to heal tissue at the cellular level. This is not the same thing as a TENS unit that is more superficial although it may feel good while it is being used. The acuscope sometimes doesn't feel like much if anything, or it can feel like a strong tingling sensation, but it is not about the sensation you feel during treatment. The effects on the tissue happen at the cellular level where the electrical currents put the cells in a functional state to heal the body. Normal healthy cells already know how to heal; that is what they do. It is when the cells are disrupted from their healthy state that they don't function as they should and cause pain and dysfunction to occur. This device may be used by different healthcare providers. It is very popular in sports medicine and recovery from injury and has been in existence for over 20 years. Unfortunately, treatment by acuscope is not very widely available. If you find a practitioner who can treat you with this, do not pass up the opportunity to try it and see if it should be a part of your Circle of Wellness.

Massage Therapist

- Bodywork includes massage as well as some other lesser known therapies like Reiki and Rolfing. Massage can support balance and relaxation by various methods used to increase blood flow and stimulate the body's own energy to heal itself. There are various levels of pressure and manipulation as well as techniques that are more energetic in nature such as Reiki. Reiki uses the healer's energy to influence the recipient's energy by different hand positions on and over the body. On the other end of the spectrum is Rolfing. It is not technically massage, but a manipulation of the soft tissue, especially the fascia, to restore balance. Fascia is a type of connective tissue that can restrict movement and function when it forms unhealthy attachments to the structures it surrounds. Like all of the other previous mentioned treatments and their providers, bodywork can be used to address TMJD specific pain and discomfort as well as to promote entire body wellness.

Body Awareness Practitioners

- Yoga, tai chi, Feldenkrais method, and Pilates. These are all different techniques used to bring awareness to your way of moving and being in your body. If you are not familiar with them, find an instructor in your area and take a class. Or ask to observe first. All the methods focus on ways to be centered, balanced, and focused in a way that seems effortless. They are not exercises in the way you may be familiar with, such as aerobics or working out at the gym to get your heart rate up and tone muscles, etc. Be aware there are hybrid workout routines that incorporate these methods, so be thoughtful and educate yourself about a class before you sign up for anything. Ideally, you want to practice as pure a form of the body awareness method that resonates with you. Try a couple or try them all and see what is right for you! It should be fun, enjoyable, and restorative.

Nutritionist/Dietician

Consider consulting with a nutritionist or dietician to find out what vitamins or other substances may be lacking in your diet that could help support your TMJ health and overall wellness. For example, anything with anti-inflammatory benefits would be a good place to start. Research nutritional supplements as there are some minerals like magnesium that play a role in reducing headaches and muscle spasms. Of course, consult your physician when considering any nutritional supplement. Just because herbs and vitamins may be natural and do not need a prescription doesn't mean they are not powerful. Be aware that nutritional supplements may have an effect on other medications or health conditions. A nutritionist or dietician would be helpful in devising a soft food menu that is nutritious and palatable. Design a custom TMJD menu for yourself that fits into your family and lifestyle. Being on a soft food diet to protect your TMJ doesn't mean it has to be all applesauce and smoothies. Get creative and find some inspiration.

Non-Physical Approaches

While you are healing the physical aspects of your body, it is important to address your mind, heart, and soul connection to your wellness. Stress counseling, therapy, meditation, and other ways to heal the mental, emotional, spiritual, and psychological aspects of your pain and dysfunction are just as important as the physical. Emotional un-wellness like heartache, anxiety, depression, and PTSD may not be the direct cause of your TMJD, but they are certainly contributing factors and most definitely are not helping your overall wellness. Use your "Wellness Journal" to help bring your awareness to these areas and seek out help and support for those areas you feel may be contributing to your un-wellness. It may sound cliché, but feelings of love and hope can do wonders to heal physical pain. There is even a study by Stanford University School of Medicine that mapped areas of the brain and showed how people in love experienced pain relief similar to prescription painkillers. How exciting is that?!

There is also an entire school of thought and study regarding the emotional connection behind physical ailments and pain in the body. Author Louise Hay wrote extensively about how illness in different areas of the body represents a corresponding emotional imbalance. It is certainly worth considering when looking at the non-physical approaches to your TMJ and overall wellness.

Explore personal development resources to enhance your ability to create the life you desire. There are countless tools to help you develop a positive mind-set. Some of my personal favorites are listed in the resources section. Find the voice that resonates with you. This is another are where guided meditation can help you focus on attracting love, health, peace, and anything you desire for your wellness. Guided meditation is a recording that you listen to that directs your thoughts and breathing to focus on that which you desire. Many are available as digital downloads you can listen to from your smartphone or computer. There is a program of recordings for balancing the connection between the left and right sides of the brain called Holosync. This is not guided meditation, but it is sort of like induced meditation as the sound waves put your brain in a meditative state. The program can help you overcome past trauma and change dysfunctional behavior. Parts of the program even allow you to record affirmations in your own voice for subliminal messages.

Self-Care: Surprise! Your Journey Begins AND Ends with YOU.

Here are suggestions for additional things you can do at home or on your own to help support your TMJ health. You can modify your diet as needed to reduce stress and strain on your TMJ. The more severe your pain and dysfunction, the softer the food, i.e., less chewing. When you are resting your TMJ due to a dislocation or other severe dysfunction, be sure to give your jaw enough time to recover. Thirty days or more may be needed before you can gradually add firmer foods. Even when you are not in a flare-up, be mindful of the food you eat and other actions that directly involve your jaw. Why put unnecessary stress on your jaw and risk making things worse? Be mindful of activities and habits that may stress your jaw. Hot or cold packs and neck wraps can help soothe when you feel sore and inflamed. Gentle stretches and exercises recommended by your physical therapist can be done daily between visits. Self-massage of tense and spasmed areas of the head and neck can also be done regularly between visits to a massage therapist. Ask your healthcare providers for advice on things you can do or avoid in your daily life to support TMJ health. You can choose how you experience being protective of your TMJ. When you think of caring for yourself and your TMJ, viewing it in a nurturing light and not as a burden can shift your entire perspective. Do you choose a path of healing and hope or a path of misery and suffering? An upward spiral is just as possible as a downward spiral.

Section 4

Destination – TMJ Health

What To Do Next?

*"Our goals can only be reached through a vehicle of a plan,
in which we must fervently believe, and upon which we must
vigorously act. There is no other route to success."*

~ Pablo Picasso

Now you know how to read the road signs and what vehicles you have to choose from as well as who your potential co-pilots will be. By now you also have a better understanding of yourself and your role as chief navigator. It's time to start creating your custom roadmap if you haven't already started doing so. Maybe you have made notes along the way. If so, gather them up and use them to help create your roadmap. It's time to plot your course! Are you excited? Nervous? Don't worry. Your roadmap is not etched in stone. You have the steering wheel! Remember, you can change course, you can revise your roadmap, you can decide which way you want to go.

I have one little surprise for you before you continue on your path to wellness. It's a little something to carry along with you on your journey that will help you stay strong and focused. When you might get confused or feel overwhelmed or want to give up, you can use this secret weapon to get through it. Take this Wellness Pledge: *I have made a committed decision to improve my TMJ health and I am fully aware that I am responsible for taking care of my body. I am improving my quality of life and I am not defined by my TMJD. I follow my roadmap with ease. No matter how difficult or challenging it may seem for a period of time, my path to well-ness is certain.* Pledge your commitment to your TMJ health and overall wellness. Write it out or print it out and post it in visible places at home, your desk at work, etc.

Let's get started. Worksheet 1

To figure out where you are now, go back to the self-assessment questions in Section 3, "Where to Begin". Your answers to those questions are your starting point. If you haven't already, take the time to write them down.

Worksheet 1 – Self-assessment, "You Are Here"

Answer the following questions from Section 3 "Where to Begin"

1) **Am I willing to take responsibility for my health?** Taking the Wellness Pledge will help you commit to this. Think about ways you do or don't take ownership of your wellness and write them down. Maybe make a list for each and see if you have more written down on one list or another. Examples of not taking ownership are: having a victim mind-set, blaming others for your health status, making excuses for not taking ownership, delaying or cancelling appointments with healthcare providers (lack of commitment and follow through), talking yourself out of taking action because "other things are more of a priority than your TMJ health". Examples of taking ownership are: taking an active role in decision making regarding treatment options for your TMJ health, educating yourself on treatment options for TMJ health and overall wellness, making and keeping appointments with healthcare providers (commitment and follow through). To really answer this question honestly, watch how you talk about your TMJD out loud as well as self-talk (that little voice inside your head).

2) **Do I listen to my body?** To help you answer this question, think about the following: How do you respond to pain and discomfort? Do you "push through the pain" thinking you can "outlast" or be "stronger" than the pain (fighting against your own body)? Do you give in to the pain thinking you "just have to live with it" (ignoring your body)? Do you ever consider what your body is trying to tell you (listening to your body)? Pain is a way of your physical body communicating important information to your brain. It is there to help us move away from the source of pain. For example, when you put your hand on a hot stove, the pain tells you to move your hand off the stove. What could your TMJD and related head and neck pain be trying to tell you? Are there more subtle signs that you are not paying attention to that occur prior to more severe pain and discomfort? There are often signs and symptoms that are overlooked that are letting you know you are nearing your threshold. Some ways to

deepen your body awareness and the mind-body connection are yoga, tai chi, Feldenkrais, and guided meditation that lead you through focusing your attention on your body from head to toe.

3) **Am I experiencing an acute flare-up, sudden onset, or am I in a chronic pain cycle?** Journaling can help you answer this question or confirm what you think is the answer. Use a Wellness Journal to track signs, symptoms, and their impact on your quality of life. One is provided in this workbook to help you get started right away.

4) **What have I done or tried already? What were the results?** Write down all treatments and/or self-care practices and whether or not they helped you. You might even rate them on a scale of 0-5. Zero being not at all and five being elimination of one or more symptoms.

1) Am I willing to take responsibility for my health?

_____

_____

_____

_____

_____

_____

_____

_____

_____

_____

_____

_____

_____

_____

_____

_____

_____

_____

_____

_____

_____

2) Do I listen to my body?

_____

_____

_____

_____

_____

_____

_____

_____

_____

_____

_____

_____

_____

_____

_____

_____

_____

_____

3) **Am I experiencing an acute flare-up, sudden onset, or am I in a chronic pain cycle?**

_____

_____

_____

_____

_____

_____

_____

_____

_____

_____

_____

_____

_____

_____

_____

_____

_____

_____

4) What have I done or tried already? What were the results?

Worksheet 2 – Keep Going

Next, to make your roadmap completely custom as it should be, think about what TMJ health means to you. What would improve your quality of life? Write them down and be as specific as possible. (Worksheet 2) Then, use those answers to set goals. It is helpful to first set short-term goals related to things such as acute pain relief. Then move on to long-term goals for chronic issues and then on to prevention of recurrence. This is due to the fact that some treatments that will get you out of immediate pain or discomfort are not long-term solutions. And some of the treatments or therapies that will help you heal long term will not immediately relieve your symptoms. For example, most people would agree that dependence on a prescription drug or drugs daily for the rest of your life is not ideal for your overall health. Therefore, while certain drugs may be helpful in the short term, so you can function and work on long-term solutions for TMJ health, they would be part of a short-term goal and not a long-term goal. When using the worksheets, remember that the goal is your desired outcome and the treatments are vehicles to help you get there. If you have difficulty putting your goals into words, you may also use images or a combination of words and images to help you envision the wellness you desire. You can use personal photos, pictures from magazines, or draw sketches if that helps you. Whatever triggers a powerful positive emotional response will be very helpful.

Once you have your starting point and goals written out, they will be helpful tools for you in at least two ways. One is to take with you to health-care provider interview appointments. Having a written list of goals to take with you to share during interview/consultation appointments will allow you to frame the conversation in terms of how a treatment or provider can and will help you move in the direction you have decided on. Having and sharing your quality of life goals will also help you and your treatment provider to be on the same page as far as expectations from any given treatment. You will be able to ask and hopefully get a satisfactory answer to questions like "Is this treatment option a solution or partial solution to a long-term goal or short-term goal? and/or "how would this treatment option impact my long-term or short-term goal?"

The second way that having your TMJ health goals written out is that you can use them as a visualization tool. If you choose to do this, and I highly recommend that you do since it is very powerful, it is very simple. Place your goals in a location where you will see them every day and spend a few minutes not only reading them, but imagining yourself living them. This is also referred to as "affirmations". I should mention here that it is very important to write your affirmations in the present tense. Avoid writing them as something you will do in the future. If you imagine them in the future, they will likely stay in the future. That is, they will always be something you are "trying to do" rather than something you "are doing". It may seem strange and unfamiliar at first, but with practice it becomes natural. Picture in your mind what that healthy TMJ image is and feel what that would be like. You can do this every step along the way by visualizing yourself having the best possible outcome from any therapy or treatment option you choose. Make it a positive experience by associating the desired results with something or someone you love. Do this regularly and repeatedly and you will reap the rewards. There are many examples of people who overcame health problems and defied their doctor's prognosis for their condition by the power of visualization. Affirmations are a daily practice to remind and assist you with visualization. By making it a daily practice and being as specific as possible, you will increase the effectiveness. In addition to visual aids and/or writing them out, there is another way to visualize your TMJ wellness goals. You can record them and listen to them repeatedly and regularly. This can be done relatively easily now with your smartphone or computer. After writing out your TMJ wellness goals, record them in the present tense as if you have already achieved them. It may take a few times to get it right as you want to really capture the feeling behind the words. You can even use certain apps to make a loop of the recording, so it continually repeats. This is really powerful when listened to right before falling asleep. Play with these different methods of visualization and see which you enjoy doing most. The ones you embrace with joy, ease, and gratitude will be those that you stick with and become a part of your path to wellness.

Worksheet 2 – "Quality of Life Goals"

1) **How do I perceive TMJD to be negatively impacting my life?** Make a list of all the ways you can think of. Section 2 "Understanding TMJ Disorder", subsection titled "Effect on Quality of Life" describes many potential ways TMJD and associated head and neck pain can negatively impact your quality of life. The list is not exclusive though; you could experience something that is not on the list. So write down anything you can think of.

2) **What would I love to do/experience that I am not doing/experiencing now due to TMJD related symptoms?** This is kind of the reverse of the first question for a reason. Have you ever heard the saying, "In the question/problem lies the answer/solution"? It's not meant to be a mind puzzle. It is an instruction. Take the list you made from question one and turn them into goals here. For example, if in question one you wrote, " I avoid eating in public and that affects my social life/family life", you can flip that around and create a goal of "I would love to be able to enjoy eating out at a restaurant with friends and family". Now you have created a quality of life goal. You can go a step further here and create an affirmation by writing "I am so happy and grateful now that I regularly enjoy eating out with friends and family (or be even more specific and insert your family's favorite restaurant name here) at _____." This is how you can create real visual imagery and emotion associated with your goal and its affirmation.

3) **Divide the quality of life goals you have set into short and long term.** You can use their importance to you (priority) to divide them. Or you can use how "easy" or "challenging" you think they will be to achieve. This is mostly a matter of perception and will be different for everyone. The length of time of some goals may be determined by certain treatments being done and taking effect. So if you know that certain treatments or procedures have a time frame for them to get results, then that will determine if they are part of a long-term goal. For example, let's say you had a goal of getting off of a pain medication. That would probably be a long-term goal because you first need to see if there is a weaning off period for the medication. Then you need

to find out by consulting your Circle of Wellness and your own research what other pain management strategies are options for you. Once you have some treatment options or therapies and practices you want to apply, write them under that quality of life goal. These are the "things" you will plug into the Roadmap Builder. You can keep following the above steps until you have a few short-term and a few long-term goals or you can start as soon as you have even one. Follow the flow chart for each treatment or practice on your list.

1) How do I perceive TMJD to be negatively impacting my life?

_____

_____

_____

_____

_____

_____

_____

_____

_____

_____

_____

_____

_____

_____

_____

_____

_____

_____

_____

_____

_____

_____

2) What would I love to do/experience that I am not doing/ experiencing now due to TMJD related symptoms?

_____

_____

_____

_____

_____

_____

_____

_____

_____

_____

_____

_____

_____

_____

_____

3) **Divide the quality of life goals you have set into short and long term.**

_____

_____

_____

_____

_____

_____

_____

_____

_____

_____

_____

_____

_____

_____

_____

_____

_____

_____

_____

_____

_____

_____

Use the Roadmap Builder

Now that you have defined where you are and where you want to go, you are ready for the next step, using the Roadmap Builder to create your custom path to wellness.

In the center of the circle, write either "me" or your name. In the surrounding radiating circles, write all the healthcare providers you are currently seeing. You can either write their actual names as in "Dr. Smith," or you can write in the practice as in "yoga" or "yoga with Jane". As you go through the process of using the Roadmap Builder, you will add or remove providers to and from your Circle of Wellness. This is another tool that can be displayed to help with visualization.

Roadmap Builder

Circle of Wellness

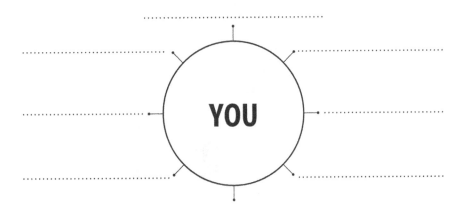

**TREATMENT I HAVE DONE/TRIED
HAS IT HELPED?**

NO   **YES**   *Add to Circle*

WHY?

Provider | Treatment not right | Need additional action/treatment

Go to interview questions. Determine if you need to locate new provider then repeat treatment. Re-evaluate.

Go to worksheet 2. re-evaluate treatment, possibly educate further on that treatment to decide if it should be used now or at all.

Go to worksheet 2. Did you fully comply? Is this treatment helped by another supportive treatment or action.

TREATMENTS NOT DONE

Research Treatment/ Locate Provider

Interview

Add to Circle **YES**   **NO**

Get treatment

Helps?

Confirm/Keep **YES**   **NO**

Why?

Provider | Treatment not right choice | Need additional treatment/ action

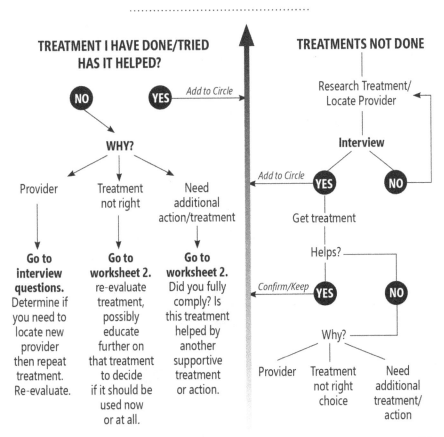

75

Circle of Wellness

Fill in your wellness information from the previous page. Continue to add your information as wellness progresses.

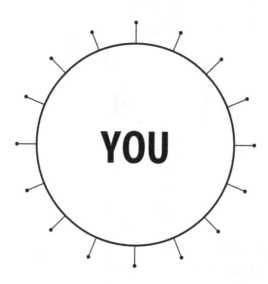

- *Dr. Jones or Yoga Class etc*
- ....
- ....
- ....
- ....
- ....
- ....
- ....
- ....

- ....
- ....
- ....
- ....
- ....
- ....
- ....
- ....
- ....

Interview Questions

Part 1

This is more of a screening process before you actually meet with the healthcare provider.

1) **Reviews:** online reviews and personal recommendations can help you get a general impression of a healthcare provider. Remember to look at the big picture and not any one single review. What common points are made by other patients? Look for the common thread.

2) **Calling an office/treatment location:** what is the first impression you get when you call there? The way the support team who handles the phone calls interacts with you says a lot about the office and provider and the experience you will have in person. Do they greet you in a caring and compassionate way? Do they treat you like a person or a "number"? Are they informed and organized? If this is somewhere you already go, do they remember you? Do they make note of your chief complaint or concern? Make clear your reason for seeking treatment there and gauge their response to that. Are they familiar with TMJD? How so? Do they follow up with your questions and concerns if they are not able to answer them at the moment?

3) **Office policies and procedures:** Do they instruct you before your appointments on what to expect and other information to prepare for your visit? This may involve things like completing forms and health history before your visits. Do they seem to have a system where everyone is on the same page? Tip: providers who have a strict cancellation policy (respect for their time) often are very organized and will respect your time more than those who are "loose" with their schedule. A provider who dedicates their undivided time to you should be appreciated.

Part 2

During your consultation or visit with provider

1) Ask, does the provider "practice what they preach"? Are they an example of the type of wellness they are providers of? For example,

does the dentist have healthy teeth and a nice smile? Would he or she undergo or have they undergone any of the treatments they recommend to you? Do they live and promote overall wellness?

2) Do they keep you waiting? Do they respect your time

3) Is the facility clean? Do they show pride in their profession by keeping it up to a certain standard of cleanliness and organization?

4) Do they acknowledge information you provided beforehand such as your chief concern or complaint? If you completed any forms or questionnaires ahead of your visit, are they addressed or incorporated now in person?

5) Do they ask you questions and listen to your answers?

6) Ask how they can help you achieve your wellness goals. What do they recommend to help you get there?

7) Repeat back treatment recommendations to get confirmation that you understand correctly.

8) Ask questions if you don't understand or need more explanation. How do they respond to your questions?

9) Ask for a printed treatment plan or recommendations. Don't be afraid or embarrassed to have information written down or spelled for you such as medications or names of procedures you are not familiar with. Don't be embarrassed to take notes. You will not be able to remember everything by memory only.

10) Be honest and as detailed and thorough as possible when providing your health history and current health status. It is better to err on the side of too much information than not enough. Something you may think has no bearing on your treatment with that provider may impact their diagnosis or recommendations.

11) Write down and ask any questions you have specific to the type of treatment they provide.

Wellness Pledge

I have made a committed decision to
improve my TMJ health and I am fully aware
that I am responsible for taking care of my body.
I am improving my quality of life and
I am not defined by my TMJD.
I follow my roadmap with ease.
No matter how difficult or challenging it may
seem for a period of time,
my path to wellness is certain.

Wellness Journal

Use these pages to track your TMJ health. For example, you can identify triggers and patterns over time. Write down when you begin or end certain therapies. You can record changes during and after treatments. You can write one thing every day that you can do to help move in the direction you want to go by saying *Today I will...* (fill in the blank).

_____

_____

_____

_____

_____

_____

_____

_____

_____

_____

_____

_____

_____

_____

_____

_____

_____

Wellness Journal

_____

_____

_____

_____

_____

_____

_____

_____

_____

_____

_____

_____

_____

_____

_____

_____

_____

_____

_____

_____

Wellness Journal

_____

_____

_____

_____

_____

_____

_____

_____

_____

_____

_____

_____

_____

_____

_____

_____

_____

_____

_____

_____

Wellness Journal

_____

_____

_____

_____

_____

_____

_____

_____

_____

_____

_____

_____

_____

_____

_____

_____

_____

_____

_____

_____

Wellness Journal

_____

_____

_____

_____

_____

_____

_____

_____

_____

_____

_____

_____

_____

_____

_____

_____

_____

_____

_____

_____

_____

_____

Wellness Journal

Wellness Journal

_____

_____

_____

_____

_____

_____

_____

_____

_____

_____

_____

_____

_____

_____

_____

_____

_____

_____

_____

_____

Wellness Journal

_____

_____

_____

_____

_____

_____

_____

_____

_____

_____

_____

_____

_____

_____

_____

_____

_____

_____

_____

_____

_____

Wellness Journal

Wellness Journal

_____

_____

_____

_____

_____

_____

_____

_____

_____

_____

_____

_____

_____

_____

_____

_____

_____

_____

_____

_____

_____

Wellness Journal

_____

_____

_____

_____

_____

_____

_____

_____

_____

_____

_____

_____

_____

_____

_____

_____

_____

_____

_____

_____

Wellness Journal

_____

_____

_____

_____

_____

_____

_____

_____

_____

_____

_____

_____

_____

_____

_____

_____

_____

_____

_____

_____

_____

_____

Wellness Journal

Wellness Journal

_____

_____

_____

_____

_____

_____

_____

_____

_____

_____

_____

_____

_____

_____

_____

_____

_____

_____

_____

_____

_____

_____

Wellness Journal

———————————————————————————

———————————————————————————

———————————————————————————

———————————————————————————

———————————————————————————

———————————————————————————

———————————————————————————

———————————————————————————

———————————————————————————

———————————————————————————

———————————————————————————

———————————————————————————

———————————————————————————

———————————————————————————

———————————————————————————

———————————————————————————

———————————————————————————

———————————————————————————

Wellness Journal

Wellness Journal

Wellness Journal

_____

_____

_____

_____

_____

_____

_____

_____

_____

_____

_____

_____

_____

_____

_____

_____

_____

_____

_____

_____

_____

Wellness Journal

_____

_____

_____

_____

_____

_____

_____

_____

_____

_____

_____

_____

_____

_____

_____

_____

_____

_____

Wellness Journal

_____

_____

_____

_____

_____

_____

_____

_____

_____

_____

_____

_____

_____

_____

_____

_____

_____

_____

_____

_____

Wellness Journal

Wellness Journal

_____

_____

_____

_____

_____

_____

_____

_____

_____

_____

_____

_____

_____

_____

_____

_____

_____

_____

_____

_____

_____

_____

Wellness Journal

Wellness Journal

Wellness Journal

Wellness Journal

_____

_____

_____

_____

_____

_____

_____

_____

_____

_____

_____

_____

_____

_____

_____

_____

_____

_____

_____

Wellness Journal

_____

_____

_____

_____

_____

_____

_____

_____

_____

_____

_____

_____

_____

_____

_____

_____

_____

_____

_____

_____

Wellness Journal

Wellness Journal

_____

_____

_____

_____

_____

_____

_____

_____

_____

_____

_____

_____

_____

_____

_____

_____

_____

_____

_____

_____

_____

Wellness Journal

Resources

Book by Louise L. Hay titled *Heal Your Body: the Mental Causes for Physical Illness and the Metaphysical Way to Heal Them.*

Article by National Institute of Health, "Facing Pain Head-On," https://www.nidcr.nih.gov/news-events/facing-pain-headon

Get the entire Workbook as a free download at
www.tmjhealthroadmap.com

A great very simple video animation of TMJ function and dysfunction, https://www.youtube.com/watch?v=QwhD5UTUW60

About the Authors

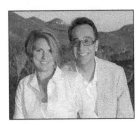

Jenna Michaud-Bonyadi is passionate about helping improve the lives of others. Her degree in Anthropology from California State University at Northridge was sparked by her combined interests in life sciences, humanity, and storytelling. Jenna has worked in several fields from English tutor to real estate broker. An avid reader with a love of writing from a young age, Jenna is excited finally to be fulfilling her life's purpose. She is blessed to have been born and raised in South Florida by a family of women who taught her to appreciate the beauty in life and who instilled in her a love of reading and encouraged her to write. Jenna currently lives on the beautiful Central Coast of California with her husband, best friend, and partner, Dino Bonyadi. They share their lives with a very large family of animals. Jenna's next book titled Unleash Your Inner Unicorn leads readers on a journey to rediscover the magic within all of us.

Dino Bonyadi, DDS, has been practicing general dentistry since graduating from the University of Southern California School of Dentistry in 1992. The creativity and artistry he brings to his dentistry extend to all areas of his life. Dino's adventurous spirit led him to take a sabbatical from his Los Angeles area practice in 2003 when he and his wife, Jenna, moved to a rural and remote but dramatic California canyon. This experience led to huge personal and professional growth as he practiced dentistry in a variety of settings and reinvented his way of life. His love of learning motivates him constantly to pursue continuing education in all areas of dentistry with a special interest in TMJD and chronic pain. Dino is inspired by nature and has always enjoyed being outdoors whether it's camping, fishing, and boating or gardening. He was at one time the largest grower in the U.S. of a rare fruit called medlar. Now he tends an orchard of heirloom figs when he is not giving five-star care to his patients in his California Central Coast private practice.

Where to buy more copies of the book:
www.tmjhealthroadmap.com

Where to get the workbook.
Available as a free download at www.tmjhealthroadmap.com

Visit Jenna's author page on FB at
https://www.facebook.com/jennamichaudbonyadiauthor

Visit Dino's practice FB page at
https://www.facebook.com/DinoBonyadiDDSFamilyDentistry

Look for the next book from Jenna Michaud-Bonyadi titled *Unleash Your Inner Unicorn* that leads readers on a journey to rediscover the magic within all of us. This book is both a personal memoir and inspirational guide for readers to live the life they were meant to live. One full of love, joy, and abundance.

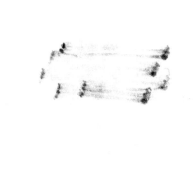

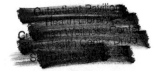

CPSIA information can be obtained
at www.ICGtesting.com
Printed in the USA
FSHW020211171220
76947FS